HERBA REMEDIES FOR GALLBLADDER:

"Revitalize Your Gallbladder Naturally"

Dr. Vera J. Reynolds

Copyright

This book is a work of non-fiction. The information, opinions, and advice presented in this book are based on the author's research and personal experience. The author and publisher make no representation or warranties with respect to the accuracy or completeness of the contents of this book and specifically disclaim any implied warranties of merchantability or fitness for a particular purpose.

The information contained in this book is provided on an "as is" basis and is intended to be used for general informational purposes only. The views and opinions expressed in this book are those of the author and do not necessarily reflect the official policy or position of any agency, organization, employer, or company.

Contents

INTRODUCTION

Deep beneath the rich fabric of our bodies lurks a little, inconspicuous organ with a vital function in our digestive system - the gallbladder. Often neglected until it raises its voice in pain and discomfort, the gallbladder silently stores and discharges bile, an essential chemical that assists in breaking down fats. When this delicate equilibrium is broken by gallstones or inflammation, it may cause agonizing agony. But worry not because the natural world provides a beautiful treasure trove of herbal medicines to alleviate gallbladder troubles, remove gallstones, and restore digestive equilibrium.

The Unsung Hero: Your Gallbladder

Before continuing our adventure into herbal therapies, it's vital to understand the gallbladder's position in our delicate digestive symphony. Nestled underneath the liver, this tiny, pear-shaped organ stores bile, a digestive fluid generated by the liver. When we ingest a meal high in fats, the gallbladder rushes into action, releasing bile into the small intestine to assist in the breakdown and absorption of lipids.

Yet, when gallstones or inflammation break this exquisite ballet, the gallbladder demands our attention.

Gallstones: Nature's Intruders

Gallstones, these little but powerful invaders, may interrupt the gallbladder's quiet life. They arise when chemicals like cholesterol and bilirubin in bile become imbalanced, producing tiny, hard deposits. These stones vary in size and may have uncomfortable symptoms, from burning pain to digestive difficulties. Conventional medicine commonly suggests gallbladder removal, but the appeal of natural options compels us to investigate the therapeutic potential of herbs.

A Herbal Renaissance: Bridging Tradition and Modernity

In recent years, herbal therapy has had a rebirth, capturing individuals seeking gentle, holistic approaches to health and well-being. Herbs, with their complicated combination of bioactive ingredients, beg us to alleviate gallbladder inflammation, remove gallstones, and foster digestive energy.

Embark on this herbal voyage with us as we dive into the exciting realm of herbal therapies for gallbladder health. These natural partners stand ready to provide consolation to a disturbed gallbladder, dissolve gallstones, and reignite the embers of digestive peace. Through centuries of traditional wisdom and the lens of modern science, these herbal companions hold the promise of renewed gallbladder vitality.

CHAPTER ONE

Understanding the Gallbladder

The gallbladder is a tiny, pear-shaped organ found underneath the liver in the human body. It performs a critical function in the digestive system by mainly acting as a reservoir for bile, a digestive fluid generated by the liver. Here are crucial points concerning the gallbladder:

1. **Anatomy:** The gallbladder is usually around 3 to 4 inches long and has a capacity of about 50 millilitres. It is in the upper right quadrant of the abdomen, tucked beneath the liver.

2. **Bile Storage:** One of the critical tasks of the gallbladder is to store and concentrate bile. Bile is needed for the digestion and absorption of dietary lipids. When we ingest fatty meals, the gallbladder contracts and discharges concentrated bile into the small intestine, where it helps emulsify fats for improved digestion.

3. **Release of Bile:** The gallbladder releases bile in response to signals from the digestive system, mainly when we consume meals containing fats. This release assists in the breakdown of lipids and enables the body to absorb the required nutrients.

4. **Regulation of Bile Flow:** The gallbladder's capacity to retain and release bile in a regulated way is vital for successful digestion. It stops a continuous bile flow into the small intestine and ensures that bitterness is accessible for fat processing.

5. **Importance in Digestion:** Without the gallbladder's participation, the digestion and absorption of lipids might be hampered, resulting in digestive pain and nutritional shortages.

In summary, the gallbladder is a tiny organ that has a crucial function in the digestive process. It stores and releases bile to help digest dietary lipids, facilitating the proper absorption of nutrients. Understanding the structure and function of the gallbladder is vital for grasping its role in maintaining overall digestive health, a subject discussed in further depth in the book "Herbal Remedies for Gallbladder."

Common Gallbladder Disorders

"Common Gallbladder Disorders" dives into many health diseases and difficulties that might affect the gallbladder. These illnesses may cause substantial pain and health issues. Here are some of the frequent gallbladder problems mentioned below:

1. **Gallstones (Cholelithiasis):** Gallstones are hardened deposits in the gallbladder. They may vary in size and produce symptoms, including severe stomach discomfort, nausea, and vomiting when they restrict the passage of bile.

2. **Gallbladder Inflammation (Cholecystitis):** Cholecystitis is the inflammation of the gallbladder, commonly caused by gallstones obstructing the cystic duct. Symptoms include muscular stomach discomfort, fever, and soreness in the upper right abdomen.

3. **Biliary Dyskinesia:** This condition includes poor gallbladder function when the gallbladder doesn't contract efficiently or adequately discharge bile.

Symptoms may include stomach discomfort, bloating, and digestive difficulties.

4. **Gallbladder Polyps:** These are growths or protrusions on the gallbladder wall. While most polyps are benign, some might be malignant. Monitoring and possibly surgical removal may be required.

5. **Choledocholithiasis:** This disorder arises when gallstones travel from the gallbladder into the common bile duct, creating an obstruction. It may lead to jaundice, pancreatitis, and extreme discomfort.

6. **Gallbladder Sludge:** Gallbladder sludge comprises thickened bile and particles that may collect in the gallbladder. While not as solid as gallstones, it may contribute to discomfort and may need treatment.

7. **Gallbladder Polyps:** These are growths or protrusions on the gallbladder wall. While most polyps are benign, some might be malignant.

Monitoring and possibly surgical removal may be required.

8. **Gallbladder Cancer:** Although uncommon, gallbladder cancer may occur. It typically remains undiscovered until it reaches an advanced stage. Symptoms may include stomach discomfort, jaundice, and unexplained weight loss.

Understanding these common gallbladder problems is vital for detecting their symptoms and finding proper medical assistance. In the book "Herbal Remedies for Gallbladder," readers may study herbal and natural techniques to treating and avoiding these diseases, supplementing traditional medical treatments where appropriate.

The Role of Herbal Remedies

"The Role of Herbal Remedies in Gallbladder Health" addresses the role of herbal remedies in preserving and increasing the well-being of the gallbladder. Here, we examine the numerous ways in which herbal therapies may significantly improve gallbladder health:

1. **Gentle Detoxification:** Herbal medicines are commonly used to help gentle detoxification of the gallbladder and liver. Certain herbs, such as milk thistle and dandelion root, are recognized for their detoxifying effects, helping to remove toxins and waste products from these organs.

2. **Anti-Inflammatory Effects:** Some plants, including turmeric and ginger, exhibit significant anti-inflammatory qualities. Inflammation may be a component of gallbladder diseases, and these herbs may help decrease inflammation and relieve related symptoms.

3. **Promoting Bile Flow:** Herbal treatments may increase bile production and encourage its healthy flow. This is especially good for persons with slow gallbladders or those at risk of gallstone production. Herbs like artichoke leaf and peppermint may aid in this process.

4. **Pain Management:** Certain herbal treatments, such as poultices and compresses, may be administered externally to decrease gallbladder pain and

discomfort. These medicines, frequently flavoured with herbs like chamomile and lavender, give comforting relief.

5. **Prevention of Gallstones:** Herbal treatments might be part of a preventative approach to gallstone development. By fostering proper digestion and a balanced diet, some herbs minimize the chance of gallstone formation.

6. **Stress Reduction:** Chronic stress may significantly impair gallbladder function. Herbal medicines like lemon balm and valerian may control pressure and induce relaxation, helping gallbladder function.

7. **Supporting Overall Digestive Health:** Many herbal medicines contribute to overall digestive health, directly connected to gallbladder function. These medicines indirectly benefit the gallbladder by boosting digestion and lowering digestive pain.

It's crucial to remember that although herbal medicines may be helpful aids in preserving gallbladder health, they should be used in combination with medical guidance and treatment, particularly in severe gallbladder diseases. Herbal therapies should be selected and given cautiously, considering individual health problems and sensitivities. The book "Herbal Remedies for Gallbladder" includes profound insights into particular herbs, formulations, and ways to support gallbladder health naturally and efficiently.

CHAPTER TWO

Herbs for Gallbladder Cleansing

Peppermint

1. Peppermint Essential Oil

Peppermint essential oil may be used topically or aromatically to enhance gallbladder health. Here's how to utilize it:

Aromatherapy:

Add a few drops of peppermint essential oil to an essential oil diffuser or a bowl of hot water. Inhale the steam to appreciate its calming scent. Peppermint's fragrance may encourage relaxation and reduce intestinal distress.

Topical Use:

Dilute a few drops of peppermint essential oil with a carrier oil (such as coconut or almond oil) and massage the mixture over your belly. Use gentle, clockwise movements to follow the route of the digestive system. This may help relax the gallbladder and decrease pain.

2. Peppermint Capsules:

Peppermint supplements in pill form are available and may be used to enhance digestive health and gallbladder function. Follow the suggested dose guidelines on the product label or check with a healthcare expert for tailored assistance.

3. Peppermint Oil Infusion:

Ingredients:

- Dried peppermint leaves
- Olive oil or another carrier oil

Instructions:

1. Fill a glass jar with dried peppermint leaves, allowing some room at the top.
2. Pour the carrier oil over the leaves until they are immersed.
3. Seal the jar securely.
4. Store the jar in a cold, dark area for approximately 2-4 weeks, stirring it gently daily to agitate the mixture.
5. After steeping, pour the oil through a fine mesh sieve or cheesecloth into a clean, dark glass container.

6. Your peppermint oil infusion is ready to use.

7. **Topical Application:** Apply the peppermint oil infusion to your belly using moderate, circular massage strokes. This may assist in relaxing the gallbladder region and alleviate pain.

Artichoke Leaf (Cynara scolymus)

1. Artichoke Leaf (Cynara scolymus)

Tinctures are concentrated herbal preparations that may be an excellent approach to employing artichoke leaf for gallbladder support. Here's how to create an artichoke leaf tincture:

Ingredients:

- Dried artichoke leaves
- High-proof alcohol (e.g., vodka or brandy)

Instructions:

1. Fill a clean glass jar with dried artichoke leaves, allowing some room at the top.

2. Pour the alcohol over the leaves until they are soaked.

3. Seal the jar securely.

4. Store the jar in a cold, dark area for approximately 2-6 weeks, stirring it gently daily to agitate the mixture.

5. After steeping, strain the liquid through a fine mesh strainer or cheesecloth into a clean, dark glass container.

6. Your artichoke leaf tincture is ready to use.

7. **Usage:** The usual dose is 30-60 drops (1-2 dropperfuls) mixed in water or juice, taken 1-3 times daily. Consult with a healthcare expert for specific dose advice.

2. Artichoke Leaf Capsules:

Artichoke leaf supplements are available in pill form and may be taken as indicated on the product label. Follow the suggested dose directions on the product label or check with a healthcare expert for tailored information.

3. Culinary Uses:

Artichoke leaves are edible and may be used in culinary preparations. Here's an essential practice:

- Fresh artichoke leaves
- Lemon juice
- Olive oil
- Salt and pepper

1. Trim the rough outer leaves of the artichoke until you reach the sensitive interior leaves.
2. Steam or boil the artichoke leaves until they become soft, generally for around 20-30 minutes.
3. Drain the leaves and let them cool.
4. Serve the artichoke leaves with a dipping sauce from lemon juice, olive oil, salt, and pepper. This may be a delightful and nutritious addition to your diet.

When utilizing artichoke leaf for gallbladder support or any other reason, it's a good idea to speak with a healthcare practitioner or herbalist, particularly if you have underlying health concerns or are taking drugs. They may give information on optimum doses and guarantee that the artichoke leaf fits your requirements.

Yellow Dock (Rumex crispus)

Here's how to make and utilize yellow dock for a gallbladder remedy:

1. Yellow Dock Tincture:

Tinctures are concentrated herbal preparations that enable you to employ yellow dock for gallbladder assistance. Here's how to create a yellow dock tincture:

Ingredients:

- Dried yellow dock root
- High-proof alcohol (e.g., vodka or brandy)

Instructions:

1. Fill a clean glass jar with dried yellow dock root, allowing some room at the top.
2. Pour the alcohol over the root until it is immersed.
3. Seal the jar securely.
4. Store the jar in a cold, dark area for approximately 2-6 weeks, stirring it gently daily to agitate the mixture.
5. After steeping, strain the liquid through a fine mesh strainer or cheesecloth into a clean, dark glass container.

6. Your yellow dock tincture is ready to use.

7. **Usage:** The usual dose is 30-60 drops (1-2 dropperfuls) mixed in water or juice, taken 1-3 times daily. Consult with a healthcare expert for specific dose advice.

2. Yellow Dock Capsules:

Yellow dock supplements are available in pill form and may be taken as indicated on the product label. Follow the suggested dose directions on the product label or check with a healthcare expert for tailored information.

3. Yellow Dock Root Infusion:

Ingredients:

Dried yellow dock root Water Instructions:

- Place dried yellow dock root in a glass jar.
- Boil water and pour it over the dried root.
- Cover the container and let it soak for several hours or overnight.
- Strain the liquid to remove the root.
- Drink the yellow dock root infusion. You may add honey or lemon for taste if desired.

This infusion might be a softer alternative to a tincture and is suitable for individuals who prefer not to ingest alcohol.

4. Yellow Dock Poultice:

A yellow dock poultice may be placed externally to the belly to reduce gallbladder pain. Here's how you prepare one:

Ingredients:

- Dried yellow dock root
- Warm water

Instructions:

1. Grind the dried yellow dock root into a fine powder.
2. Mix the powder with enough warm water to make a thick, paste-like consistency.
3. Apply the paste directly to the belly, over the gallbladder region.
4. Cover with a clean towel or bandage and let it on for around 20-30 minutes.
5. Remove the poultice and rinse the area with warm water.

Chicory (Cichorium intybus)

Here's how to make and utilize chicory for a gallbladder remedy:

1. Chicory Tincture:

Tinctures are concentrated herbal preparations that enable you to employ chicory for gallbladder assistance. Here's how to create a chicory tincture:

Ingredients:

- Dried chicory root
- High-proof alcohol (e.g., vodka or brandy)

Instructions:

1. Fill a clean glass jar with dried chicory root, allowing some room at the top.
2. Pour the alcohol over the root until it is immersed.
3. Seal the jar securely.
4. Store the jar in a cold, dark area for approximately 2-6 weeks, stirring it gently daily to agitate the mixture.
5. After steeping, strain the liquid through a fine mesh strainer or cheesecloth into a clean, dark glass container.

6. Your chicory tincture is ready to use.

7. **Usage:** The usual dose is 30-60 drops (1-2 dropperfuls) mixed in water or juice, taken 1-3 times daily. Consult with a healthcare expert for specific dose advice.

2. Chicory Capsules:

Chicory supplements are available in pill form and may be taken as indicated on the product label. Follow the suggested dose directions on the product label or check with a healthcare expert for tailored information.

3. Chicory Root Infusion:

Ingredients:

Dried chicory root Water Instructions:

1. Place dried chicory root in a glass jar.

2. Boil water and pour it over the dried root.

3. Cover the container and let it soak for several hours or overnight.

4. Strain the liquid to remove the root.

5. Drink the chicory root infusion. You may add honey or lemon for taste if desired.

This infusion might be a softer alternative to a tincture and is suitable for individuals who prefer not to ingest alcohol.

4. Chicory Leaf Salad:

4. Chicory Leaf Salad:

Chicory leaves are edible and may be used in salads. Here's how to cook a simple chicory leaf salad:

Ingredients:

- Fresh chicory leaves
- Olive oil
- Lemon juice
- Salt and pepper

Instructions:

1. Wash and dry the chicory leaves.
2. Tear the leaves into bite-sized pieces.
3. Drizzle olive oil and lemon juice over the leaves.
4. Season with salt and pepper to taste.
5. Toss the salad and serve as a side dish or appetizer.
6. Chicory leaves have a somewhat bitter taste and may offer a distinctive flavour to your salads.

Barberry (Berberis vulgaris)

Here are some different methods to utilize barberry for gallbladder support:

1. Barberry Tincture:

Tinctures are concentrated herbal extracts that may be used to enhance gallbladder health. Here's how to create a barberry tincture:

Ingredients:

- Dried barberry root or bark
- High-proof alcohol (e.g., vodka or brandy)

Instructions:

1. Fill a clean glass jar with dried barberry root or bark, allowing some room at the top.
2. Pour the alcohol over the root or bark until it is immersed.
3. Seal the jar securely.
4. Store the jar in a cold, dark area for approximately 2-6 weeks, stirring it gently daily to agitate the mixture.

5. After steeping, strain the liquid through a fine mesh strainer or cheesecloth into a clean, dark glass container.
6. Your barberry tincture is ready to use.
7. **Usage:** The usual dose is 30-60 drops (1-2 dropperfuls) mixed in water or juice, taken 1-3 times daily. Consult with a healthcare expert for specific dose advice.

2. Barberry Capsules:

Barberry supplements are available in pill form and may be taken as indicated on the product label. Follow the suggested dose directions on the product label or check with a healthcare expert for tailored information.

3. Barberry Extract:

You may also acquire liquid barberry extracts, commonly accessible at health food shops. Follow the dosing directions on the product packaging.

4. Barberry Poultice:

A barberry poultice may be administered externally to the gallbladder region to reduce pain. Here's how you prepare one:

- Dried barberry root or bark
- Warm water

1. Grind the dried barberry root or bark into a fine powder.
2. Mix the powder with enough warm water to make a thick, paste-like consistency.
3. Apply the paste directly to the belly, over the gallbladder region.
4. Cover with a clean towel or bandage and let it on for around 20-30 minutes.
5. Remove the poultice and rinse the area with warm water.
6. Use this poultice as required for relief from gallbladder pain.

Globe Artichoke (Cynara cardunculus var. scolymus)

Here's how to prepare and utilize globe artichoke for gallbladder support:

Globe artichoke extract is a concentrated version of the plant that may be used to enhance gallbladder health. You may get it at health food shops or cook it yourself if you can access fresh globe artichokes. Here's how to produce an extract:

Ingredients:

- Fresh globe artichokes

Instructions:

1. Start with fresh globe artichokes. Remove the stiff outer leaves and chop the artichoke hearts into tiny pieces.
2. Place the chopped artichoke hearts in a glass container.
3. Pour a high-proof alcohol (e.g., vodka or brandy) over the artichoke pieces until they are immersed.
4. Seal the jar securely.
5. Store the jar in a cold, dark area for approximately 2-6 weeks, stirring it gently daily to agitate the mixture.
6. After steeping, strain the liquid through a fine mesh strainer or cheesecloth into a clean, dark glass container.
7. Your globe artichoke extract is ready to use.

8. **Usage:** The usual dose is 30-60 drops (1-2 dropperfuls) mixed in water or juice, taken 1-3 times daily. Consult with a healthcare expert for specific dose advice.

2. Globe Artichoke Capsules:

Globe artichoke supplements are available in pill form and may be taken as indicated on the product label. Follow the suggested dose directions on the product label or check with a healthcare expert for tailored information.

3. Globe Artichoke in Cooking:

Globe artichokes are edible and may be used in numerous culinary preparations. They may be steamed, boiled, roasted, or sautéed. Artichoke hearts may be a great addition to salads, spaghetti, or as a side dish. Consuming globe artichokes as part of your daily diet might give possible gallbladder assistance.

4. Globe Artichoke Juice:

You may also create a fresh globe artichoke juice to ingest. Combine new artichoke hearts with water, drain the concoction, and drink the juice. This might be a more solid but bitter choice for gallbladder support.

Oregon Grape (Mahonia aquifolium)

Here's how to prepare and utilize Oregon grape for gallbladder support:

1. Oregon Grape Tincture:

Tinctures are concentrated herbal preparations that enable you to employ Oregon grapes for gallbladder assistance. Here's how to create an Oregon grape tincture:

Ingredients:

- Dried Oregon grape root or bark
- High-proof alcohol (e.g., vodka or brandy)

Instructions:

1. Fill a clean glass jar with dried Oregon grape root or bark, allowing some room at the top.
2. Pour the alcohol over the root or bark until it is immersed.
3. Seal the jar securely.
4. Store the jar in a cold, dark area for approximately 2-6 weeks, stirring it gently daily to agitate the mixture.

5. After steeping, strain the liquid through a fine mesh strainer or cheesecloth into a clean, dark glass container.

6. Your Oregon grape tincture is ready to use.

7. **Usage:** The usual dose is 30-60 drops (1-2 dropperfuls) mixed in water or juice, taken 1-3 times daily. Consult with a healthcare expert for specific dose advice.

2. Oregon Grape Capsules:

Oregon grape supplements are available in pill form and may be taken as instructed on the product label. Follow the suggested dose directions on the product label or check with a healthcare expert for tailored information.

3. Oregon Grape Extract:

You may also purchase liquid Oregon grape extracts, commonly accessible at health food shops. Follow the dosing directions on the product packaging.

4. Oregon Grape Poultice:

To decrease pain, an Oregon grape poultice may be administered topically to the gallbladder region. Here's how you prepare one:

- Dried Oregon grape root or bark
- Warm water

1. Grind the dried Oregon grape root or bark into a fine powder.
2. Mix the powder with enough warm water to make a thick, paste-like consistency.
3. Apply the paste directly to the belly, over the gallbladder region.
4. Cover with a clean towel or bandage and let it on for around 20-30 minutes.
5. Remove the poultice and rinse the area with warm water.
6. Use this poultice as required for relief from gallbladder pain.

Ginger (Zingiber officinale)

Ginger is recognized for its digestive and anti-inflammatory characteristics, which might be helpful for gallbladder health. Here are some other ways to utilize ginger:

1. Ginger Capsules:

Ginger supplements in pill form are readily available and may be taken as advised on the product label. Follow the suggested dose directions on the product label or check with a healthcare expert for tailored information.

2. Ginger Tincture:

You may create a ginger tincture to use as a gallbladder treatment. Here's how you prepare it:

Ingredients:

- Fresh ginger root
- High-proof alcohol (e.g., vodka or brandy)

Instructions:

1. Wash and peel a fresh ginger root.
2. Slice or slice the ginger root into tiny pieces.
3. Fill a clean glass jar with the chopped ginger, allowing some room at the top.
4. Pour the alcohol over the ginger until it is immersed.
5. Seal the jar securely.
6. Store the jar in a cold, dark area for approximately 2-6 weeks, stirring it gently daily to agitate the mixture.

7. After steeping, strain the liquid through a fine mesh strainer or cheesecloth into a clean, dark glass container.

8. Your ginger tincture is ready to use.

9. **Usage:** The usual dose is 30-60 drops (1-2 dropperfuls) mixed in water or juice, taken 1-3 times daily. Consult with a healthcare expert for specific dose advice.

3. Ginger Poultice:

A ginger poultice may be placed externally to the belly to reduce gallbladder pain. Here's how you prepare one:

Ingredients:

- Fresh ginger root
- Warm water

Instructions:

1. Grate or finely chop fresh ginger to yield roughly 2-3 teaspoons of ginger pulp.

2. Mix the ginger pulp with warm water to produce a paste.

3. Apply the paste directly to the belly, over the gallbladder region.

4. Cover with a clean towel or bandage and let it on for around 20-30 minutes.

5. Remove the poultice and rinse the area with warm water.

6. Use this poultice as required for relief from gallbladder pain.

Fennel (Foeniculum vulgare)

Fennel is recognized for its digestive characteristics, which might be excellent for gallbladder health. Here are some other ways to utilize fennel:

1. Fennel Capsules:

Fennel supplements in pill form may be taken as indicated on the product label. Follow the suggested dose directions on the product label or check with a healthcare expert for tailored information.

2. Fennel Tincture:

You may create a fennel tincture to use as a gallbladder treatment. Here's how you prepare it:

Ingredients:

- Crushed fennel seeds

- High-proof alcohol (e.g., vodka or brandy)

1. Fill a clean glass jar with crushed fennel seeds, allowing some room at the top.
2. Pour the alcohol over the crushed seeds until they are soaked.
3. Seal the jar securely.
4. Store the jar in a cold, dark area for approximately 2-6 weeks, stirring it gently daily to agitate the mixture.
5. After steeping, strain the liquid through a fine mesh strainer or cheesecloth into a clean, dark glass container.
6. Your fennel tincture is ready to use.
7. **Usage:** The usual dose is 30-60 drops (1-2 dropperfuls) mixed in water or juice, taken 1-3 times daily. Consult with a healthcare expert for specific dose advice.

3. Fennel Poultice:

A fennel poultice may be placed externally to the belly to reduce gallbladder pain. Here's how you prepare one:

Ingredients:

- Crushed fennel seeds

- Warm water

1. Crush fennel seeds to yield around 2-3 teaspoons of crushed seeds.
2. Mix the crushed seeds with warm water to produce a paste.
3. Apply the paste directly to the belly, over the gallbladder region.
4. Cover with a clean towel or bandage and let it on for around 20-30 minutes.
5. Remove the poultice and rinse the area with warm water.
6. Use this poultice as required for relief from gallbladder pain.

Milk Thistle Capsules

Milk thistle supplements are available in pill form and may be taken as indicated on the product label. Typically, a usual dose is 250-500 mg of standardized milk thistle extract (containing 70-80% silymarin) taken 1-3 times a day, depending on the usage purpose. Be careful to follow the suggested dose on the product box or check with a healthcare expert for individualized assistance.

Milk Thistle Tincture:

Ingredients:

- Dried milk thistle seeds
- High-proof alcohol (e.g., vodka or brandy)

Instructions:

1. Fill a clean glass jar with dried milk thistle seeds, allowing some room at the top.
2. Pour the alcohol over the seeds until they are soaked.
3. Seal the jar securely.
4. Store the jar in a cold, dark area for 2-4 weeks, stirring it gently daily to agitate the mixture.
5. After steeping, strain the liquid through a fine mesh strainer or cheesecloth into a clean, dark glass container.
6. Your milk thistle tincture is ready to use. The usual dose is 20-30 drops (1-2 dropperfuls) mixed in water, juice, or tea, taken 1-3 times daily. Be careful to contact a healthcare expert for individualized dose advice.

When utilizing milk thistle pills or preparations, it's vital to check with a healthcare professional or herbalist, particularly if you have underlying health concerns, are pregnant or breastfeeding, or are taking drugs. They can assist with the optimum dose and guarantee that milk thistle fits your unique requirements.

Dandelion Root Tincture:

Ingredients:

- Dried dandelion root
- High-proof alcohol (e.g., vodka or brandy)

Instructions:

1. Fill a clean glass jar with dried dandelion root, allowing some room at the top.
2. Pour the alcohol over the root until it is immersed.
3. Seal the jar securely.
4. Store the jar in a cold, dark area for 2-6 weeks, stirring it gently daily to agitate the mixture.
5. After steeping, strain the liquid through a fine mesh strainer or cheesecloth into a clean, dark glass container.

6. Your dandelion root tincture is ready to use.

7. The usual dose is 30-60 drops (1-2 dropperfuls) diluted in water, juice, or tea, taken 1-3 times daily.

8. Consult with a healthcare expert for specific dose advice.

2. Dandelion Root Capsules:

Dandelion root supplements are available in pill form and may be taken as indicated on the product label. Typical doses may vary, so follow the suggested dosage guidelines on the product box or speak with a healthcare expert for tailored counsel.

3. Roasted Dandelion Root with Coffee:

Ingredients:

- Dandelion roots (washed, dried, and cut)
- Baking sheet
- Oven

Instructions:

1. Preheat your oven to 350°F (175°C).

2. Wash the dandelion roots well, wiping away any debris.

3. Chop the dandelion roots into tiny, uniform pieces.

4. Spread the chopped roots in a single layer on a baking sheet.

5. Roast the roots in the oven for approximately 2 hours or until they turn dark and coffee-like in colour.

6. Remove from the oven and allow them to cool fully.

7. Grind the roasted dandelion roots to a coarse powder using a coffee grinder, mortar, and pestle.

8. Store the roasted dandelion root coffee replacement in an airtight container.

9. Brew it as regular coffee by adding hot water and steeping for a few minutes.

10. You may add your choice of sweeteners, milk, or cream.

4. Culinary Uses:

You may integrate fresh or dried dandelion root in culinary preparations. For example, add cleaned, chopped, and roasted dandelion roots to salads, soups, or stir-fries for their earthy taste and possible health benefits.

When utilizing dandelion root for any reason, speaking with a healthcare practitioner or herbalist is good, particularly if you have underlying health concerns or are taking drugs. They may give information on optimum doses and guarantee that dandelion root fits your unique requirements.

Turmeric Paste:

- ¼ cup of ground turmeric
- ½ cup of water
- ½ teaspoon of black pepper (optional, but increases absorption)

1. In a small saucepan, mix the ground turmeric and water.
2. Heat the mixture over low to medium heat, stirring regularly until it forms a thick paste. This usually takes approximately 7-10 minutes.
3. If desired, add black pepper to the mixture and combine thoroughly.
4. Allow the paste to cool, then transfer it to an airtight container.
5. You may use this turmeric paste as a basis for numerous dishes, such as curries, stews, and golden milk (turmeric latte).
6. It's an easy method to integrate turmeric into your everyday diet.

Turmeric supplements are available in pill form and may be taken as indicated on the product label. Typical doses may vary, so follow the suggested dosage guidelines on the product box or speak with a healthcare expert for tailored counsel.

Turmeric is a versatile spice that may be utilized in numerous savoury cuisines. It gives a warm, earthy taste and vivid yellow colour to meals. You may use turmeric in:

1. **Curries and stir-fries:** Add turmeric powder to your favourite curry or stir-fry dishes.
2. **Rice dishes:** Mix turmeric into rice to produce tasty turmeric rice.
3. **Soups and stews:** Enhance the taste and colour of soups and stews with a bit of turmeric.
4. **Roasted veggies:** Sprinkle turmeric over roasted vegetables like cauliflower or carrots before baking.

Turmeric paste may also be used topically for its possible skin advantages. Here's how you prepare it:

Ingredients:

- One tablespoon of turmeric powder
- 1-2 teaspoons of yoghurt or honey (for a creamy consistency)

Instructions:

1. Mix the turmeric powder with yoghurt or honey to produce a thick mixture.
2. Apply the paste to your skin and keep it on for around 10-15 minutes.
3. Rinse off with warm water.

This turmeric face mask may aid with skin lightening and minimizing the appearance of blemishes. However, conduct a patch test before applying it to your face since turmeric may discolour the skin momentarily.

When using turmeric in any form, be mindful that it may stain surfaces, clothes, and skin. Also, speak with a healthcare professional or herbalist, particularly if you have underlying health concerns or are taking drugs since turmeric may mix with certain medications or have contraindications in some instances.

CHAPTER THREE

Herbal Teas for Gallbladder Support

Peppermint Tea

Ingredients:

- 1-2 tablespoons of dried peppermint leaves or one peppermint tea bag
- 1 cup of hot water

Instructions:

1. Boil a cup of water and let it cool slightly for a minute or two so it's not boiling.
2. Place the dried peppermint leaves in a tea infuser or straight into a cup if you're using a tea bag.
3. Pour the heated water over the peppermint leaves or tea bag.
4. Cover the cup with a lid or saucer and steep it for 5-10 minutes. The longer you steep it, the greater the taste will be.
5. Remove the tea infuser or tea bag.
6. Optionally, you may add honey or lemon for taste, but keeping it basic for gallbladder support is better.

7. Enjoy your peppermint tea leisurely. Sip it when it's still warm but not burning hot.

Peppermint tea is renowned for its ability to soothe the digestive system, perhaps aiding with gallbladder pain. However, speaking with a healthcare expert if you have particular gallbladder concerns or other medical disorders is crucial to confirm that peppermint tea suits your circumstances.

Dandelion Root Tea

Here's how to create dandelion root tea for gallbladder support:

Ingredients:

- 1-2 tablespoons of dried dandelion root or one dandelion root tea bag
- 1 cup of hot water

Instructions:

1. Boil a cup of water and let it cool slightly for a minute or two so it's not too hot.

2. Place the dried dandelion root in a tea infuser or straight into a cup if you're using a tea bag.

3. Pour the heated water over the dandelion root or tea bag.

4. Cover the cup with a lid or saucer and steep it for 5-10 minutes. The longer you steep it, the greater the taste will be.

5. Remove the tea infuser or tea bag.

6. You may sip the tea as is or add honey or lemon for taste, but it's best to keep it simple for gallbladder support.

7. Enjoy your dandelion root tea when it's still warm but not burning hot.

Dandelion root is known to enhance liver and gallbladder function by boosting the generation and flow of bile.

Milk Thistle Tea

Milk thistle tea is widely used for gallbladder support owing to its possible liver-protective characteristics, which may indirectly assist the gallbladder. Here's how to create milk thistle tea for gallbladder support:

Ingredients:

- 1-2 tablespoons of crushed milk thistle seeds or one milk thistle tea bag
- 1 cup of hot water

Instructions:

1. Boil a cup of water and let it cool slightly for a minute or two so it's not boiling.
2. Place the crushed milk thistle seeds in a tea infuser or straight into a cup if you're using a tea bag.
3. Pour the heated water over the milk thistle seeds or tea bag.
4. Cover the cup with a lid or saucer and steep it for 5-10 minutes. The longer you steep it, the greater the taste will be.
5. Remove the tea infuser or tea bag.
6. You may drink the milk thistle tea as is or add honey or lemon for taste.
7. Enjoy your milk thistle tea when it's still warm but not burning hot.

Milk thistle is renowned for its capacity to maintain and promote liver function, which may influence the gallbladder as the liver and gallbladder work closely together in the digestive process. However, you should contact a healthcare practitioner before drinking milk thistle tea for gallbladder support, particularly if you have specific gallbladder concerns or other medical disorders. If you encounter any ill effects, cease usage and seek medical assistance.

Artichoke Leaf Tea

Artichoke leaf tea enhances gallbladder health by boosting bile production and facilitating digestion. Here's how to create artichoke leaf tea for gallbladder support:

Ingredients:

- 1-2 tablespoons of dried artichoke leaves or one artichoke leaf tea bag
- 1 cup of hot water

Instructions:

1. Boil a cup of water and let it cool slightly for a minute or two so it's not boiling.
2. Place the dried artichoke leaves in a tea infuser or straight into a cup if you're using a tea bag.

3. Pour the heated water over the artichoke leaves or tea bag.

4. Cover the cup with a lid or saucer and steep it for 5-10 minutes. The longer you steep it, the greater the taste will be.

5. Remove the tea infuser or tea bag.

6. You may sip the artichoke leaf tea as is or add honey or lemon for taste if preferred.

7. Enjoy your artichoke leaf tea when it's still warm but not burning hot.

Artichoke leaves are known to support good digestion and encourage bile flow, which might assist the gallbladder. However, if you have particular gallbladder concerns or other medical conditions, it's advised to contact a healthcare practitioner before drinking artichoke leaf tea for gallbladder support. If you encounter any ill effects, cease usage and seek medical assistance.

Turmeric Tea

Turmeric tea might be a helpful alternative for gallbladder support owing to its anti-inflammatory qualities. Here's how to create turmeric tea for gallbladder support:

Ingredients:

- One teaspoon of powdered turmeric or 1-2 slices of fresh turmeric root
- 1 cup of hot water
- A sprinkle of black pepper (optional, although it may boost turmeric's potency)

Instructions:

1. Boil a cup of water and let it cool slightly for a minute or two so it's not boiling.
2. Place the ground turmeric or fresh turmeric slices in a cup.
3. Pour the heated water over the turmeric.
4. If you're using fresh turmeric, you may add a sprinkle of black pepper to boost the absorption of turmeric's active ingredient, curcumin.
5. Stir well and let the tea infuse for around 5-10 minutes. The longer you steep it, the greater the taste will be.
6. Remove the turmeric slices or filter the tea if you use ground turmeric.
7. Enjoy your turmeric tea when it's still warm but not burning hot.

Turmeric is recognized for its anti-inflammatory and antioxidant characteristics, which may help decrease inflammation in the gallbladder and improve overall digestive health. However, if you have particular gallbladder concerns or other medical conditions, it's advised to contact a healthcare practitioner before drinking turmeric tea for gallbladder assistance. If you encounter any ill effects, cease usage and seek medical help.

Ginger Tea

Ginger tea may be a calming and helpful option for gallbladder health owing to its digestive and anti-inflammatory characteristics. Here's how to create ginger tea for gallbladder support:

Ingredients:

- 1-2 tablespoons of freshly grated ginger or ginger slices (approximately a 1-inch chunk)
- 1 cup of hot water
- Honey or lemon (optional, for flavoring)

1. Boil a cup of water and let it cool slightly for a minute or two so it's not boiling.
2. Place the freshly grated ginger or ginger slices in a cup.
3. Pour the heated water over the ginger.
4. Optionally, you may add honey or lemon for taste, but it's better to keep it basic for gallbladder support.
5. Stir well and let the tea infuse for around 5-10 minutes. The longer you steep it, the stronger the ginger taste will be.
6. Remove the ginger slices or drain the tea if you use grated ginger.
7. Enjoy your ginger tea when it's still warm but not burning hot.

Ginger is recognized for improving digestion, lowering inflammation, and calming the digestive system, perhaps benefitting the gallbladder. However, if you have particular gallbladder concerns or other medical conditions, it's advised to contact with a healthcare practitioner before consuming ginger tea for gallbladder assistance. If you encounter any ill effects, cease usage and seek medical assistance.

Lemon Balm Tea

Lemon balm tea is a pleasant herbal choice that may assist gallbladder health owing to its calming effects. Here's how to create lemon balm tea for gallbladder support:

Ingredients:

- 1-2 tablespoons of dried lemon balm leaves or one lemon balm tea bag
- 1 cup of hot water

Instructions:

1. Boil a cup of water and let it cool slightly for a minute or two so it's not boiling.
2. Place the dried lemon balm leaves in a tea infuser or straight into a cup if you're using a tea bag.
3. Pour the heated water over the lemon balm leaves or tea bag.
4. Cover the cup with a lid or saucer and steep it for 5-10 minutes. The longer you steep it, the greater the taste will be.
5. Remove the tea infuser or tea bag.
6. Enjoy your lemon balm tea as is. Lemon balm has a lovely, mild, lemony taste on its own.

Yellow Dock Root Tea

Yellow dock root tea is a herbal infusion produced from the roots of the yellow dock plant (Rumex crispus). This tea is often used for its possible health advantages, including digestive support and as a mild laxative. While it's not often connected with gallbladder support, it may assist overall digestion, thereby aiding the gallbladder.

Here's how to create yellow dock root tea:

Ingredients:

- 1-2 tablespoons of dried yellow dock root or one yellow dock root tea bag
- 1 cup of hot water
- Honey or lemon (optional, for flavoring)

Instructions:

1. Boil a cup of water and let it cool slightly for a minute or two so it's not boiling.
2. Place the dried yellow dock root in a tea infuser or straight into a cup if you're using a tea bag.
3. Pour the heated water over the yellow dock root or tea bag.

4. Optionally, you may add honey or lemon for taste, but it's better to keep it simple for this tea.

5. Stir well and let the tea infuse for around 5-10 minutes. The longer you steep it, the greater the taste will be.

6. Remove the tea infuser or tea bag.

7. Enjoy your yellow dock root tea when warm but not burning hot.

Chicory Root Tea

Chicory root tea is not generally connected with gallbladder support, but it is recognized for its possible digestive advantages, which may indirectly assist to overall digestive health, including gallbladder function. Chicory root contains inulin, a soluble fibre that may improve digestion and maintain a healthy gut microbiota.

Here's how to create chicory root tea:

Ingredients:

- 1-2 tablespoons of dried chicory root or one chicory root tea bag
- 1 cup of hot water

1. Boil a cup of water and let it cool slightly for a minute or two so it's not boiling.
2. Place the dried chicory root in a tea infuser or straight into a cup if you're using a tea bag.
3. Pour the heated water over the chicory root or tea bag.
4. Stir well and let the tea infuse for around 5-10 minutes. The longer you steep it, the greater the taste will be.
5. Remove the tea infuser or tea bag.
6. Enjoy your chicory root tea as is. Chicory root has a somewhat bitter and earthy taste.

Barberry Root Bark Tea

Barberry root bark tea is not a generally known herbal medicine for gallbladder support, but it includes berberine, an alkaloid that may have potential advantages for digestion and liver health. Berberine is recognized for its anti-inflammatory and antibacterial qualities, which may indirectly assist the gallbladder and general digestive health.

Here's how to create barberry root bark tea:

- 1-2 tablespoons of dried barberry root bark or one barberry root bark tea bag
- 1 cup of hot water

1. Boil a cup of water and let it cool slightly for a minute or two so it's not boiling.
2. Place the dried barberry root bark in a tea infuser or straight into a cup if you're using a tea bag.
3. Pour the heated water over the barberry root bark or tea bag.
4. Stir well and let the tea infuse for around 5-10 minutes. The longer you steep it, the greater the taste will be.
5. Remove the tea infuser or tea bag.
6. Enjoy your barberry root bark tea when warm but not burning hot.

CHAPTER FOUR

Creating Herbal Tinctures and Extracts

Herbal Extraction Methods

Herbal extraction techniques include collecting bioactive chemicals from medicinal plants or herbs for different applications, including medical, culinary, or cosmetic benefits. These approaches seek to extract the necessary phytochemicals while reducing contaminants and conserving the herb's medicinal effects. Here are some typical herbal extraction methods:

1. Infusion:

- Infusion is the process of steeping dried or fresh herbs in hot water.
- Typically used for fragile sections of plants including leaves, blossoms, and soft stems.
- Common for creating herbal teas.
- The water removes water-soluble components from the botanicals.

2. **Decoction:**

- Decoction involves boiling more problematic plant elements like roots, bark, and seeds in water.
- This approach is used to extract chemicals that need higher temperatures for extraction.
- The resultant liquid is more concentrated than an infusion.

3. **Maceration:**

- Maceration is a cold extraction procedure where plants are steeped in a solvent like alcohol or oil.
- The solvent removes both water-soluble and lipid-soluble molecules.
- Commonly used for creating herbal tinctures.

4. **Percolation:**

- Percolation is a more complex extraction procedure widely employed in herbal medicine manufacture.
- It involves gently running a solvent through a bed of plants to extract chemicals.
- This approach is efficient and provides for greater control of the extraction process.

5. Cold Pressing:

- Cold pressing produces essential oils from fragrant plant components, such as citrus peels.
- It involves applying mechanical pressure to the plant material without utilizing heat.
- The extracted oil is highly concentrated and keeps its smell.

6. Steam Distillation:

- Steam distillation is a typical technique for obtaining essential oils from fragrant plants.
- Steam is poured through the plant material, causing the essential oils to evaporate and condense into a separate container.
- This approach is excellent for volatile, heat-sensitive chemicals.

7. Solvent Extraction:

- Solvent extraction includes employing organic solvents like ethanol or hexane to extract different phytochemicals from plant material.
- It is widely employed for acquiring complicated chemicals and is anticipated in the manufacturing of herbal extracts and supplements.

8. **Supercritical Fluid Extraction (SFE):**

- SFE is a sophisticated approach employing supercritical carbon dioxide (CO_2) as a solvent.

- CO_2 is pushed to a supercritical state, which enables it to behave as both a liquid and a gas, efficiently removing chemicals without leaving solvent residues.

- This process is very selective and is used for extracting certain chemicals.

9. **Enfleurage:**

- Enfleurage is an old procedure used to extract aromatic chemicals from flowers.

- It includes putting petals in a layer of odourless fat or oil to absorb the aroma.

- Repeatedly changing the petals enables for the absorption of aromatic chemicals, which are subsequently separated from the fat or oil.

The choice of extraction process relies on the kind of herb, the desired components, and the intended application of the extract. Each approach has benefits and drawbacks, and herbalists, pharmacists, and manufacturers chose the most acceptable method depending on these variables. Quality control and safety issues are also crucial when utilizing plant extracts for medical or nutritional reasons.

Recipe: Gallbladder Detox Tincture

A gallbladder cleansing tincture may be produced using a mix of herbs known to assist gallbladder health. This tincture is designed to be taken in tiny, regulated dosages, so it's vital to check with a healthcare expert before taking it, particularly if you have specific gallbladder concerns or other medical disorders. Here's a basic recipe for a gallbladder detox tincture:

Ingredients:

- 1 part dandelion root (Taraxacum officinale)
- 1 part milk thistle seeds (Silybum marianum)
- 1 part turmeric root (Curcuma longa)
- 1 part ginger root (Zingiber officinale)
- 80-proof vodka or brandy (enough to cover the herbs

Instructions:

1. Prepare the Herbs:

- If using fresh herbs, cut them coarsely.

- If using dried herbs, measure them according on the "parts" you've determined. For example, if you're using 1 cup as 1 part, you'll need 1 cup of each herb.

2. **Combine the Herbs:**

   - Mix all the prepared herbs in a clean glass container.

3. **Add Alcohol:**

   - Pour enough 80-proof vodka or brandy over the herbs to thoroughly cover them. Ensure there's an additional inch or two of liquid for the herbs to absorb part of it.

4. **Seal the Jar:**

   - Seal the jar securely with a lid.

5. **Shake and Store:**

   - Shake the container carefully to ensure the herbs are well soaked with the alcohol.
   - Store the sealed jar in a cold, dark area for approximately 4-6 weeks. Shake the pot lightly every day or so to stir the mixture.

6. Strain the Tincture:

- After the steeping time, strain the liquid through a fine mesh strainer or cheesecloth into a clean, dark glass container.
- Squeeze the herbs to remove any leftover juice.

7. Label the Bottle:

- Label the bottle with the tincture's name, components, and the date it was prepared.

8. Usage:

- Consult a healthcare practitioner for customized dose advice, since tinctures vary in Potency.
- Typically, tinctures are taken in dropperfuls (20-40 drops) diluted in water or juice 1-3 times day.
- Start with a lesser dosage and gradually raise it as required while watching for unwanted effects.

Please note that herbal treatments should be taken with carefully and under the advice of a healthcare expert, particularly if you have certain health issues or are using pharmaceuticals. This gallbladder detox tincture is not a replacement for medical therapy, and its efficacy might vary from person to person.

Dosage and Safety Guidelines

When utilizing herbal treatments, especially tinctures, it's vital to follow dose and safety requirements to guarantee their efficacy and avoid possible hazards. Here are some basic dose and safety considerations for utilizing herbal remedies:

1. Consult a Healthcare Professional:

Before beginning any herbal therapy, particularly if you have underlying medical issues, are pregnant or breastfeeding, or are on medicines, visit a trained healthcare expert. They can give specialized assistance depending on your individual scenario.

2. Start with Low Dosages:

Begin with the lowest advised dose for the herbal cure and watch your body's reaction. You may gradually raise the dose as required.

3. Follow Label Instructions:

If utilizing commercial herbal items, such as tinctures or supplements, carefully read and follow the dose directions on the product label.

4. Understand Potency:

Herbal medicines vary in Potency dependent on herb kind, preparation technique, and concentration. Be cautious of the Potency of the therapy you are applying.

5. Monitor for Adverse Effects:

Pay attention to how your body responds to the herbal cure. If you encounter any ill effects, cease usage and seek medical assistance.

6. Be Consistent:

Take herbal treatments constantly as suggested. Some drugs may need consistent usage over time to get the intended effects.

7. Be Patient:

Herbal medicines may take time to provide apparent benefits. Be patient and give ample time for the therapy to work.

8. Interactions and Contraindications:

Be mindful of possible interactions between herbs and drugs you are taking. Some plants may interact with prescription medicines and have contraindications for particular medical conditions.

9. Avoid Overuse:

Avoid overusing herbal therapies, since excessive usage may lead to unwanted consequences or impaired efficacy.

10. Quality Matters:

Use high-quality herbs and herbal items from reliable suppliers to guarantee purity and Potency.

11. Rotate Herbs:

If you take herbal medicines for a lengthy time, consider rotating herbs or taking breaks to avoid tolerance or possible negative effects.

12. Stay Hydrated:

Drinking enough of water may assist flush out toxins and boost the body's natural detoxification processes while utilizing herbal medicines.

13. Keep Records:

Keep a note of the herbs you take, doses, and any affects or changes in your health. This information might be important for your healthcare practitioner.

14. Children and Elderly:

Be careful while utilizing herbal medicines for children and the elderly, since their doses may vary from those of adults. Consult with a healthcare practitioner for help.

CHAPTER FIVE

Gallbladder-Friendly Diet and Nutrition

Foods to Avoid for Gallbladder Health

Maintaining a healthy gallbladder generally includes adopting dietary decisions that support its function and avoid the development of gallstones or gallbladder disorders. Here are items to avoid or restrict for gallbladder health:

1. **Rich-Fat meals:** Avoid or restrict meals rich in harmful saturated and trans fats, since they might promote the production of extra bile, possibly leading to gallbladder pain. Examples include fried meals, fatty meats, and processed snacks.

2. **Processed meals:** Highly processed and packaged meals generally include harmful fats, additives, and preservatives that may stress the gallbladder. Opt for complete, unprocessed foods wherever feasible.

3. **Fried meals:** Fried meals are often rich in harmful fats and may be tough for the gallbladder to handle. Choose culinary techniques like baking, grilling, or steaming instead.

4. **Spicy Foods:** Spicy foods, particularly the gallbladder, might irritate the digestive system. If you discover that spicy meals produce pain, try lowering your consumption.

5. **Full-Fat Dairy Products:** Whole milk, full-fat cheeses, and creamy dairy products may be rich in saturated fat. Opt for lower-fat or dairy-free options if you're sensitive to greasy meals.

6. **Red Meat:** Red meat, particularly fatty slices, may be hard to digest and may contribute to gallbladder inflammation. Choose lean cuts of meat or alternate protein sources like chicken, fish, or plant-based proteins.

7. **Refined Sugars and Sugary Beverages:** Excessive sugar consumption may lead to obesity, a risk factor for gallstone development. Limit sugary

meals and beverages, especially sodas, sweets, and desserts.

8. **rich-Cholesterol Foods:** Foods rich in cholesterol may lead to developing cholesterol gallstones. Reduce your consumption of egg yolks, organ meats, and high-cholesterol dairy items.

9. **Caffeine:** While moderate caffeine use is usually regarded safe, individuals may find caffeine exacerbates gallbladder pain. Pay attention to how your body responds, and try lowering caffeine if required.

10. **Alcohol:** Excessive alcohol intake may affect the liver and lead to gallbladder troubles. If you prefer to consume alcohol, do it in moderation and speak with your healthcare professional.

11. **Quick Weight reduction Diets:** Crash diets or quick weight reduction programs that entail significant calorie restriction might raise the risk of gallstones. Aim for moderate, sustained weight reduction if required.

12. **Low-Fiber Diets:** Low-fiber diets may lead to gallstone development. To promote digestive health, incorporate lots of high-fiber foods such fruits, vegetables, whole grains, and legumes.

13. **Large Meals:** Overeating or ingesting enormous meals may overburden the gallbladder, resulting to pain. Practice portion management and eat smaller, more frequent meals if required.

Remember that individual dietary sensitivities might vary, and what provokes gallbladder pain in one person may not effect another. Suppose you have particular gallbladder difficulties or worries. In such scenario, it's essential to talk with a healthcare expert or a qualified dietitian who can give specific nutritional advice depending on your individual condition.

Foods that Support Gallbladder Function

Maintaining a healthy gallbladder entails adopting dietary decisions that support its function and avoid the development of gallstones or other disorders. Here are foods that may aid gallbladder health:

1. **Fiber-Rich meals:** High-fiber meals, such as fruits, vegetables, whole grains, and legumes, may help regulate digestion and avoid constipation. Fibre binds to cholesterol and helps prevent the production of cholesterol gallstones.

2. **Lean Proteins:** Opt for lean protein sources including chicken, fish, tofu, and lentils. These proteins are more accessible for the gallbladder to digest than fatty beef cuts.

3. **Healthy Fats:** Include sources of healthy fats in your diet, such as avocados, nuts, seeds, and olive oil. These fats are less likely to produce gallbladder pain than saturated and trans fats.

4. **Omega-3 Fatty Acids:** Fatty fish like salmon, mackerel, and trout are rich in omega-3 fatty acids, which have anti-inflammatory effects and may improve gallbladder health.

5. **Fruits and veggies:** Consume a range of colourful fruits and veggies. These foods include critical nutrients, antioxidants, and fibre that help overall digestive health.

6. **Low-Fat Dairy:** If you prefer dairy, go for low-fat or non-fat varieties of milk, yoghurt, and cheese. These are lower in saturated fat, which might be gentler on the gallbladder.

7. **Citrus Fruits:** Citrus fruits including lemons, oranges, and grapefruits are rich in vitamin C and may help prevent gallstones by lowering the likelihood of cholesterol accumulation in the gallbladder.

8. **Herbs and Spices:** Incorporate herbs and spices like turmeric, ginger, peppermint, and rosemary into your cuisine. These plants may have anti-inflammatory and digestive properties.

9. **Whole Grains:** Choose grains like brown rice, quinoa, oats, and whole wheat over processed

grains. Whole grains give greater fibre and minerals that assist digestive health.

10. **Water:** Staying hydrated is vital for general health and may help avoid gallstone development. Aim to drink an appropriate quantity of water throughout the day.

11. **Apple Cider Vinegar:** Some feel that apple cider vinegar may assist support good digestion and minimize the chance of gallstone development. You may dilute it with water and drink it before meals.

12. **Coffee:** Moderate coffee drinking has been related with a lower incidence of gallstone development in several studies. However, individual reactions to coffee might differ.

13. **Artichokes:** Artichokes include chemicals that may increase bile synthesis and assist gallbladder function. Include artichokes in your diet, either cooked or as a salad.

14. **Beets:** Beets are high in betaine, which may improve liver and gallbladder function. You may consume beets roasted, in salads, or as a juice.

Remember that a balanced diet that includes a range of nutrient-rich foods is vital for general health, including gallbladder health. Maintaining a healthy weight via a balanced diet and frequent physical exercise helps minimize the chance of gallstone development. Suppose you have particular gallbladder difficulties or worries. In such scenario, it's essential to talk with a healthcare expert or a qualified dietitian who can give specific nutritional advice depending on your individual condition.

Incorporating Herbs into Your Diet

Incorporating herbs into your diet may be a delightful and wholesome way to enrich your meals while benefitting from their possible medical effects. Here are some recommendations on how to integrate herbs into your regular diet:

1. **Fresh Herbs:** Fresh herbs are fragrant and vivid in taste. They work nicely in salads, sauces, and

garnishes for numerous cuisines. Common fresh herbs include basil, parsley, cilantro, mint, and dill.

2. **Dried Herbs:** Dried herbs are handy and have a longer shelf life. They are ideal for flavoring soups, stews, marinades, and roasted meats. Some dried herbs include oregano, thyme, rosemary, and sage.

3. **Herbal Teas:** Herbal teas are a simple way to experience the benefits of herbs. You may buy herbal tea mixes or create your own by steeping dried herbs like chamomile, peppermint, or lavender. Enjoy them hot or cold.

4. **Infused Oils and Vinegar:** Create flavoured oils and vinegar by infusing them with herbs.
Place fresh herbs in a clean, dry container, add the oil or vinegar, and let it rest for a few weeks to build taste.
Use these for salad dressings or sprinkling over foods.

5. **Smoothies:** Add fresh or dried herbs to your smoothies for a distinctive flavor. Mint, basil, and

parsley may provide freshness to fruit and vegetable smoothies.

6. **Herb-Infused Water:** Enhance simple water by adding fresh herbs and slices of citrus fruits like lemon or lime. It's a pleasant and healthful alternative to sugary drinks.

7. **Herb-Infused Butter:** Mix fresh or dried herbs into melted butter to produce herb-infused butter. Use it as a savory spread for toast or a topping for grilled veggies.

8. **Herb Pesto:** Mix fresh herbs, garlic, nuts, olive oil, and Parmesan cheese. Use it as a sauce for spaghetti, a marinade for meats, or a dip for bread.

9. **Herb-Rubbed Meats:** Create herb rubs by mixing dried herbs, garlic powder, and other ingredients. Rub the mixture onto meats before grilling, roasting, or pan-searing.

10. **Herb-Infused Salt:** Mix dry herbs with salt to produce herb-infused salt. Use it as a spice for different foods to enhance depth of taste.

11. **Herbal Salsas:** Make herbal salsas using fresh herbs, tomatoes, onions, and spices. They accompany grilled meats, seafood, and tacos.

12. **Herbal Soups:** Add fresh herbs like basil, cilantro, or parsley to homemade soups and stews before serving to improve the tastes.

13. **Herb-Seasoned Rice and Grains:** Mix chopped fresh herbs into cooked rice, quinoa, or couscous for a herbal spin on your side dishes.

14. **Herbal Marinades:** Create marinades for meats and tofu by blending herbs with olive oil, citrus juice, and seasonings. Let the ingredients marinate for additional taste.

15. **Herbal Garnishes:** Use fresh herbs as a garnish to add colour and taste to your cuisine. Sprinkle chopped herbs over salads, soups, and main dishes.

Remember that herbs not only improve the flavor of your food but may also give health advantages. Experiment with various spices to discover which tastes and combinations you appreciate best while enjoying their potential health benefits.

CHAPTER SIX

Managing Gallstone Pain Naturally

Easing Pain with Herbal Poultices

Herbal poultices may be a supplementary way to assist alleviate gallstone discomfort, while they are not a replacement for medical therapy or intervention. Gallstone discomfort may be severe, so visit a healthcare expert for an appropriate diagnosis and treatment plan. If your healthcare physician permits the use of herbal poultices, here's how you can prepare and apply one:

Ingredients:

- **Dried or fresh herbs:** Some herbs that may be good for gallstone discomfort are ginger, turmeric, and chamomile.
- **Water or carrier:** When blended with the spices, you'll need enough water to make a paste-like consistency.

1. **Select the Herbs:**

- Choose one or more herbs recognized for their anti-inflammatory and calming effects. Ginger and turmeric are widely used for digestive difficulties, while chamomile may aid with inflammation and pain.

2. **Prepare the Herbs:**

- If using fresh herbs, coarsely cut or smash them to release their juices and medicinal ingredients.
- If utilizing dried herbs, you may either use them as-is or produce a powder by grinding them.

3. **Mix with Water or Carrier:**

- Gradually add water (or a suitable carrier like olive oil) to the herbs, stirring until you create a thick, paste-like consistency.
- Ensure the mixture is moist enough to spread readily but not unduly runny.

4. Apply the Poultice:

- Spread the herbal mixture evenly onto a clean, thin cloth or gauze. Fold the cloth half to make a "sandwich" with the poultice in the centre.

5. Apply to the Abdomen:

- Place the poultice immediately on the abdomen region where you are feeling gallstone discomfort. Ensure that the skin is clean and dry before application.

6. Cover and Secure:

- Cover the poultice with a clean towel or plastic wrap to prevent it from drying out. You may secure it in place using a bandage or wrap.

7. Leave in Place:

- Allow the poultice to rest on the skin for around 20-30 minutes to an hour. You may modify the length dependent on your comfort level and the herb used.

8. Remove and Cleanse:

- Gently remove the poultice and wash the area with warm water to eliminate any residue.

- You may repeat the poultice application as frequently as required, depending on the severity of pain and the herb utilized.

Tips:

- Be careful when applying poultices on delicate or injured skin, since certain plants may irritate.
- Always conduct a patch test with any herbal combination before applying it to a wider area.
- While herbal poultices may ease gallstone discomfort, they should not substitute medical examination and treatment for gallstones.

Herbal Compresses for Gallbladder Pain

Herbal compresses may be a calming and natural approach to ease gallbladder discomfort, while they are not a substitute for medical therapy if you suspect gallbladder disorders. If you feel severe or chronic pain, obtaining medical help for a correct diagnosis and treatment plan is vital. Here's how to prepare and utilize herbal compresses for gallbladder discomfort:

- **Dried or fresh herbs:** Some herbs that may be good for gallbladder discomfort are chamomile, ginger, and mint.
- Clean cloth or gauze
- Hot water

Instructions:

1. Select the Herbs:

   - Choose one or more herbs recognized for their calming and anti-inflammatory effects.
   - Chamomile is relaxing, ginger may aid with digestion and inflammation, and mint has a cooling effect.

2. Prepare the Herbs:

   - If utilizing fresh herbs, coarsely cut or smash them to release their active ingredients.
   - If utilizing dried herbs, you may either use them as-is or produce a powder by grinding them.

3. Create a Herbal Infusion:

   - Boil water and pour it over the picked herbs in a heatproof basin or container.

- Allow the herbs to soak in the boiling water for around 5-10 minutes, making a firm herbal infusion.

4. Soak the Cloth:

- Immerse a clean towel or gauze in the herbal infusion. Make sure it's damp but not leaking.

5. Squeeze Out Excess Liquid:

- Gently compress the moistened cloth to remove any extra liquid, leaving it damp.

6. Apply the Compress:

- Lie down in a comfortable posture.
- Place the moist herbal compress on the region of your abdomen where you are suffering gallbladder discomfort.
- Cover the compress with plastic wrap to maintain warmth and moisture.

7. Leave in Place:

- Allow the herbal compress to stay in place for around 20-30 minutes. Relax and breathe deeply at this period.

8. Repeat as Needed:

- You may repeat the herbal compress application as frequently as required to ease pain. You may also alternate between hot and cold compresses if it is comforting.

Tips:

- Be careful with the temperature of the herbal infusion. Ensure it's pleasantly heated and not too hot to cause burns.

- Always conduct a patch test with any herbal combination before applying it to a wider skin area to ensure you don't have an allergic response or skin sensitivity to the herbs.

While herbal compresses may temporarily reduce gallbladder pain, they should not substitute medical examination and treatment for gallbladder disorders. If you experience severe or chronic pain, visit a healthcare practitioner.

Yoga and Breathing Exercises

Yoga and breathing exercises may be important tools for maintaining general well-being and may help ease some of the pain associated with gallbladder disorders. However, it's vital to speak with a healthcare practitioner before beginning any new workout or yoga practice, particularly if you have specific gallbladder issues. Here are some yoga positions and breathing techniques that may be beneficial:

Yoga Poses:

Child's Pose (Balasana):

- Kneel on the floor, sit back on your heels, and extend your arms forward, lowering your chest toward the ground.
- This position may help relax and stretch the abdomen region, thereby alleviating pain.

Cat-Cow Stretch (Marjaryasana-Bitilasana):

- Start on your hands and knees in a tabletop posture.
- Inhale as you arch your back, raising your head and tailbone (Cow Pose).
- Exhale as you circle your back, tucking your chin and tailbone (Cat Pose).
- This mild flow may assist improve spine flexibility and facilitate digestion.

Seated Forward Bend (Paschimottanasana):

- Sit with your legs out in front of you.

- Inhale to extend your spine, then exhale as you tilt at your hips to reach forward toward your toes.

- This position may assist reduce stress in the abdomen region.

- Lie on your back with your legs bent.

- Gently rotate your knees to one side while maintaining your shoulders on the ground.

- This twist might assist with digestion and ease stress in the belly.

- Lie on your back with your legs bent and feet flat on the floor.

- Inhale and raise your hips off the ground, forcing your feet and shoulders into the mat.

- Bridge Pose may assist improve digestion and decrease pain.

Deep Belly Breathing:

- Sit or lay down in a comfortable posture.
- Place one hand on your chest and the other on your abdomen.
- Inhale deeply through your nose, allowing your belly to rise as you fill your lungs.
- Exhale gently through your mouth, allowing your abdomen to descend.

This deep breathing method may improve relaxation and reduce stress.

Diaphragmatic Breathing:

- Sit comfortably with one hand on your chest and the other on your abdomen.
- Inhale deeply through your nose, concentrating on extending your diaphragm and allowing your abdomen to rise.
- Exhale gently through your mouth, allowing your abdomen to descend.
- Diaphragmatic breathing may aid with stress reduction and relaxation.

- Sit in a comfortable cross-legged stance.

- Close your right nostril with your right thumb and inhale through your left nose.

- Close your left nostril with your proper ring finger, release your right nose, and exhale.

- Inhale via your right nostril, shut it with your thumb, release your left nostril, and exhale.

- This method is thought to balance energy and induce calm.

Yoga and breathing techniques may be effective for controlling stress, fostering relaxation, and boosting general well-being. However, they should be utilized as supplementary practices with proper medical care and counseling. Always visit a healthcare expert for individualized suggestions, particularly if you have specific gallbladder concerns or significant discomfort.

CHAPTER SEVEN

Preventing Gallbladder Problems

Lifestyle Tips for Gallbladder Health

Maintaining gallbladder health is vital for general well-being and digestive comfort. Here are some lifestyle practices that maintain gallbladder health:

Maintain a Healthy Weight:

- Achieving and maintaining a healthy weight via a balanced diet and regular exercise will help lower the chance of gallstone development.

Eat a Balanced Diet:

- Consume a diet rich in fruits, vegetables, whole grains, lean proteins, and healthy fats. Avoid excessive intake of high-fat and high-cholesterol foods.

- Practice portion control to avoid overeating, which may stress the gallbladder. Eating smaller, more frequent meals may also be useful.

Stay Hydrated:

- Drink lots of water throughout the day to improve overall digestion and help avoid gallstones.

Fiber-Rich Foods:

- Include high-fiber foods including fruits, vegetables, whole grains, and legumes. Fibre may assist regulate digestion and minimize the risk of gallstones.

Limit Processed Foods:

- Minimize intake of processed and fried meals, generally rich in harmful fats and chemicals that might stress the gallbladder.

Choose Healthy Fats:

- Opt for healthy fats like avocados, almonds, seeds, and olive oil while avoiding saturated and trans fats.

- If you consume alcohol, do it in moderation, since excessive alcohol use may affect the liver and gallbladder.

- Regular physical exercise, such as brisk walking, running, or cycling, helps maintain a healthy weight and promote overall digestion.

- Chronic stress may disrupt digestion and may lead to gallbladder pain. Practice stress-reduction strategies like yoga, meditation, or deep breathing exercises.

- Crash diets or quick weight reduction programs that entail significant calorie restriction might increase the risk of gallstone development. Aim for moderate, sustained weight reduction if required.

- If you have particular gallbladder difficulties or a family history of gallstones, visit a healthcare expert for counseling and frequent check-ups.

Stay Informed:

- Educate yourself on gallbladder health and possible risk factors, particularly if you have a family history of gallbladder difficulties.

Follow Medical Advice:

- If you've been diagnosed with gallbladder disease or have had gallbladder-related pain, follow your healthcare provider's treatment and dietary advice.

Post-Surgery Care:

- If you've had your gallbladder removed (cholecystectomy), follow your healthcare provider's post-surgery advice, which may include dietary adjustments.

Remember that preserving gallbladder health is part of an overall healthy lifestyle. It's vital to contact with a healthcare expert if you encounter chronic or severe gallbladder-related symptoms, since they can give specific guidance and suggestions based on your individual condition.

Exercise and Physical Activity

Exercise and physical exercise are key components of a healthy lifestyle, and they may contribute to gallbladder health by helping to maintain a healthy weight and improving overall digestion. Here are some fitness and physical activity guidelines to maintain gallbladder health:

Regular Aerobic Exercise:

Engage in frequent aerobic exercises such brisk walking, running, swimming, cycling, or dancing. As health recommendations urge, strive for at least 150 minutes of moderate-intensity aerobic exercise or 75 minutes of vigorous-intensity aerobic activity every week.

1. Strength Training:

Incorporate strength training activities into your program to develop and maintain muscular mass. Strength exercise may enhance metabolism and help weight control.

2. Core Strengthening:

Include activities that target the core muscles, such as planks, bridges, and abdominal exercises. A strong core may assist in correct posture and digestion.

3. Flexibility and Stretching:

Stretching activities like yoga or Pilates may increase flexibility and aid with posture, which can favorably benefit digestive comfort.

4. Low-Impact Activities:

If you have joint concerns or prefer low-impact exercise, try sports like swimming, water aerobics, or stationary cycling.

5. Daily Movement:

Incorporate physical exercise into your everyday life by climbing the stairs, walking or cycling for transportation, and standing or moving about during lengthy periods of sitting.

6. Posture Awareness:

Pay attention to your posture, which might assist in appropriate digestion. Avoid slouching and practice sitting and standing with a straight back.

7. Breathing Exercises:

Incorporate deep breathing exercises and relaxation methods into your routine to alleviate stress, which may influence digestion.

8. Stay Hydrated:

Drink water before, during, and after exercise to keep hydrated and help overall digestion.

9. Warm-Up and Cool Down:

Always warm up before intensive activity and cool down afterwards to avoid injuries and improve healthy circulation.

10. Consult a Healthcare Professional:

If you have particular gallbladder difficulties or a history of gallbladder troubles, visit a healthcare physician or a physical therapist for exercise advice suited to your circumstances.

Remember that consistency is key when it comes to exercise and physical activity. Start with activities you love and progressively increase the intensity and time as your fitness level increases. If you have any medical ailments or concerns, contact with a healthcare practitioner before starting a new fitness regimen to confirm that it is safe and suitable for your circumstances.

Stress Management Techniques

Stress management is critical for general health, including gallbladder health, since prolonged stress may disrupt digestion and lead to pain. Here are some stress management practices that may help you decrease tension and increase well-being:

1. Deep Breathing Exercises:

Practice deep breathing methods, such as diaphragmatic breathing or the 4-7-8 method. These exercises may help relax the nervous system and lessen tension.

2. Meditation & Mindfulness:

Engage in regular meditation or mindfulness techniques to raise awareness of your thoughts and emotions and decrease stress. You may utilize guided meditation applications or attend meditation courses.

3. Yoga and Tai Chi:

Both yoga and Tai Chi combine physical movement with awareness and deep breathing, making them great stress management methods.

4. Progressive Muscle Relaxation:

Learn gradual muscle relaxation methods to reduce muscular tension and promote calm.

5. Mindful Eating:

Practice mindful eating by savouring each meal, chewing gently, and paying attention to your body's hunger and fullness signals. Avoid eating when preoccupied or anxious.

6. Regular Exercise:

Engage in regular physical activity, such as aerobic exercise, weight training, or yoga, to produce endorphins and relieve stress.

7. Adequate Sleep:

Prioritize excellent sleep to help your body to heal and better handle stress. Create a nighttime routine and keep a regular sleep pattern.

8. Social Support:

Connect with friends and loved ones, and express your thoughts and worries. A robust social support network may bring emotional comfort and stress alleviation.

9. Time Management:

Organize your duties and prioritize obligations to prevent emotions of overload. Break complex activities into smaller, achievable chunks.

10. Set Boundaries:

Establish reasonable limits in your personal and professional life to avoid overextending yourself and enduring unneeded stress.

11. Engage in Relaxation Activities:

Participate in calming hobbies like reading, bathing, listening to soothing music, or spending time in nature.

12. Journaling:

Keep a diary to communicate your ideas and feelings. Writing may be a therapeutic technique to process stress and gain perspective.

13. Professional Help:

If stress becomes unbearable or persistent, consider obtaining support from a mental health professional or therapist.

14. Biofeedback and Relaxation Techniques:

Explore biofeedback and relaxation methods that help you acquire control over physiological reactions to stress, such as heart rate and muscular tension.

15. Positive Affirmations:

Use positive affirmations to reframe negative ideas and build a more optimistic mentality.

16. Limit Stressors:

Identify causes of stress in your life and take actions to lessen or eliminate them wherever feasible. This may require establishing limits or making modifications in your regular routine.

Remember that various tactics work for other individuals, so investigating and discovering the stress management solutions that connect with you is crucial. Consistently adopting these activities into your everyday life will help decrease stress, promote gallbladder health, and contribute to overall well-being.